EXERCISE THE GENTLE WAY WITH CHAIR YOGA FOR SENIORS

Mercy Marley

Disclaimer

Table of contents

INTRODUCTION
Why Is Chair Yoga for Seniors Such an Effective Form of Exercise?
Is Chair Yoga Challenging Enough to Be Effective?
Why Doing Yoga on a Chair Is Beneficial for Seniors
Make Sleeplessness, Arthritis, and Constipation Much Easier to Manage or Even Eliminate
Why Not Begin Doing Some Relaxing Chair Yoga Right This Very Minute?
Is It True That Only Old People Can Do Chair Yoga?
How to Get Started with Relaxing Chair Yoga and What You Need to Get Started
There Is No Such Thing as the "Right" or "Wrong" Kind of Yoga to Practice at Your Age
Conclusion

INTRODUCTION

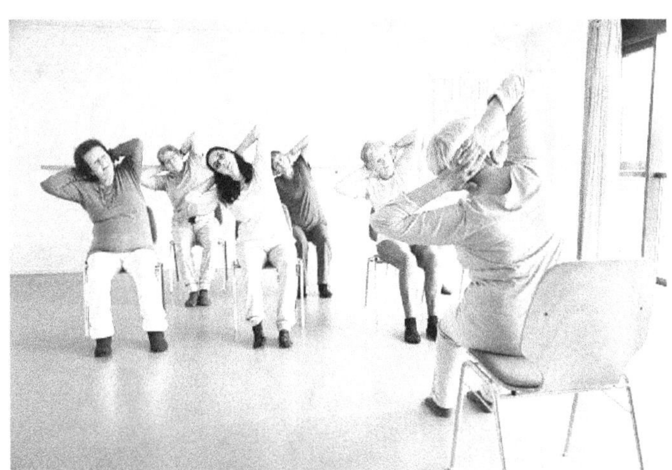

You are in for a real treat if you have never before experienced the advantages that chair yoga for seniors can provide. Over the course of the last several years, I've developed an addiction to this simple but effective exercise. I really hope that sharing my enthusiasm for chair yoga may inspire you to give it a try.

Exercising regularly is essential to maintaining a healthy and active lifestyle, which becomes more crucial as we get older. On the other hand, many people in their golden years may suffer from physical restrictions that prohibit them from partaking in conventional kinds of exercise. A solution to this problem is offered by chair yoga, which is a low-impact, gentle type of physical exercise that can easily be adapted to cater to the specific requirements of each individual participant.

Chair yoga is a subgenre of yoga in which a chair is used as a support for various yoga poses. Because of this, chair yoga is a kind of exercise that is suitable for older people and those who have mobility issues. In addition to the many positive effects it may have on your mind and emotions, it can help you become more flexible, enhance your balance, and boost your total physical strength.

Chair yoga helps to alleviate tension, anxiety, and discomfort while fostering relaxation and a general feeling of well-being. This is accomplished via a series of mild stretches, deep breathing exercises, and mindfulness practices. Because it is a secure and efficient type of exercise that can be conducted in the comfort of your own home, it is a great alternative for seniors who may have difficulties leaving their house or taking part in activities that involve a group of people.

Chair yoga is ideal for elderly citizens because of its versatility and low-impact nature, making it the ideal form of exercise for those looking to improve their health without running the risk of injury or strain. No matter how much experience you have with yoga or how new you are to the practice, this kind of physical activity may be modified to match your specific requirements and objectives, allowing you to feel your very best and enjoy life to the fullest.

Mercy Marley

Why Is Chair Yoga for Seniors Such an Effective Form of Exercise?

It is likely that you will have walked two million steps by the time you become 60 years old. If you are like the majority of us, you have undoubtedly also experienced your fair share of physical harm, whether in the form of injuries or diseases. It's possible that you've had your hip replaced. Or maybe, like me, you have endured a fractured ankle (or two).

As we approach our 60s, we are acutely aware of the critical need of maintaining a healthy level of physical fitness and flexibility. However, the majority of us just cannot stand going to gyms and doing aerobics lessons.

The question now is, what are the other options? The moderate kind of yoga that is practiced by many of the ladies I know is turning out to be an excellent alternative for getting back into shape beyond the age of 60. But what if you have trouble moving about or if you simply feel like you're becoming older and more fragile? It's possible that it's time to start thinking about chair yoga.

Is Chair Yoga Challenging Enough to Be Effective?

Now I know what you're going through in your head. "I don't see how sitting in a chair could possibly count as exercise." I can attest to the effectiveness of chair yoga on the basis of my personal practice, and I must say that I was very impressed by its benefits. The best part is that since it is so simple to get to, it is the type of physical activity that you will choose to do each and every day.

Mercy Marley

Why Doing Yoga on a Chair Is Beneficial for Seniors

The fact of the matter is that everyone, regardless of age, inflexibility, or even handicap, may benefit from practicing yoga. A common proverb among yoga instructors goes something like this: "If you can breathe, you can perform some sort of yoga."
Chair yoga is a great alternative for those who are unable to participate in conventional mat yoga because they are unable to get down on the floor. The following is a short list of the several advantages that may be gained by practicing yoga while seated on a chair:

Experience Relaxation
Very few individuals pause to consider that the ability to relax is a talent that can be learned. We have a propensity to believe that the conditions of our life are too stressful and, as a result, we are unable to relax.

Learning how to relax properly is a talent that, like any other, can be developed through repeated practice. A qualified teacher of chair yoga will begin by instructing you in yoga breathing techniques, which are useful not only during the session but also outside of it, whenever you feel the need to relax and unwind.

Improve Flexibility

Some individuals have the misconception that becoming older automatically results in a reduction of flexibility. This is a common misunderstanding. The concept of "use it or lose it" is really how flexibility works in practice. Flexibility is a skill that may be developed at any age. People who begin practicing yoga when they are in their 60s, 70s, 80s, or even 90s often discover that they recover flexibility in their muscles, joints, and connective tissues as a result.

Those who practice yoga consistently over an extended period of time claim not only that they restore lost mobility but also that they often become more limber than they were in their earlier years.

Make Sleeplessness, Arthritis, and Constipation Much Easier to Manage or Even Eliminate

The majority of people who try chair yoga say that after one to three months of consistently attending courses once a week, it helps them sleep better at night. Chair yoga has helped a good number of senior students who previously struggled with chronic constipation to enjoy more regular bowel movements without the need of medicine. Yoga has been shown to be effective in reducing or eliminating pain from a variety of illnesses, including but not limited to arthritis, sciatica, chronic backache, and even certain headaches.

Don't let excuses prevent you from giving your body the love and attention it so richly deserves.

Let's be honest. When it comes to beginning a fitness regimen, especially one as simple and non-intimidating as chair yoga, we may come up with dozens upon dozens of reasons why we just can't get started. It's possible that you, just like I have, have put on a few more pounds during the last year. Or, it's that you simply feel rigid and unyielding.

It's possible that you've hurt yourself. Another possibility is that you believe you are "too busy" to engage in physical activity. These are not objections to chair yoga; on the contrary, they are all arguments in favor of giving it a try.

Before beginning any kind of fitness routine, you should make it a point to consult with your primary care physician first. This is due to the fact that everyone has a unique physical make-up. Having said that, I have never encountered a single person who has disliked beginning gentle yoga, particularly chair yoga. I believe this to be the case.

The advantages to one's body are just part of the story. Reconnecting with your body and finding mental peace may also be accomplished via the practice of chair yoga.

You may Find That Chair Yoga Is Just What You Need to Boost Your Confidence

To tell you the truth, when I first began taking regular yoga courses, I discovered that I was too tense and rigid to really enjoy the practice of doing yoga. It seemed as if I lacked the flexibility and balance to do even the most fundamental of asanas (movements). As a result, I became disheartened. Even just sitting in a cross-legged stance was difficult for me even though I wanted to perform the positions correctly.Instead of giving up completely, as I may have in the past, I made the decision to participate in chair yoga courses instead. Wow! What a dramatic change! Simply being able to lean on the chair for support helped me address a lot of the flexibility and confidence problems that I had been struggling with. I'm at the point where I can start incorporating some additional easy yoga postures into my regimen.

Why Not Begin Doing Some Relaxing Chair Yoga Right This Very Minute?

If the thought of beginning a new yoga program gives you butterflies, I want you to know that I totally get where you're coming from and that I empathize with the way you feel. I, too, had such thoughts and feelings.

You can find a ton of free chair yoga classes on YouTube, and most of them are designed to be done in the comfort of your own home. Don't be discouraged if you don't like the first thing you try; instead, look for a different instructor and give it another shot.

You can also participate in chair yoga, which is offered at some senior centers; therefore, if you want to do it with your friends, investigate what options are available in your community. You could also try inviting some of your friends over to your house so that you can all participate in an online chair yoga session together.

Is It True That Only Old People Can Do Chair Yoga?

I gradually came to the realization that chair yoga isn't just for elderly people, despite the fact that elderly people can certainly gain advantages from the additional support. Everyone may participate in chair yoga. In point of fact, given that baby boomers spend the majority of their time sedentary, one might make the case that we are in most need of it.

Since you are going to be seated anyhow, you may as well take advantage of the situation.

Sitting for long periods of time is one of the risks that come with contemporary living. According to a number of studies, sitting for lengthy periods of time may potentially be just as detrimental to your health as smoking. Setting an alarm to remind yourself to get up and go for a walk once per hour is one possible solution to this problem. In addition, including chair yoga into your daily practice can assist in maintaining the lubrication of your joints and the pliability of your body.

Why not include some chair yoga into your everyday practice, seeing as how you are currently seated there? Your joints, muscles, and tendons will all be grateful to you. And when you're in a good mood, you'll find that you have more energy to get things done.

How to Get Started with Relaxing Chair Yoga and What You Need to Get Started

One Chair

Instead of selecting a seat that compels you to slump and lean back, go for one that puts your shoulders in front of your hips and puts you in a position where you can sit up straight. In an ideal situation, you should choose a chair that does not have armrests or one that is sufficiently broad so that there is a space of several inches between your body and the armrests.

The use of a Strap or Belt

If you already have a yoga strap, you are more than welcome to use it. In the event that you do not own one, you may use a lengthy belt, such as the one found on a bathrobe. If you want to, you may even borrow the leash that you use for your dog.

A Massive or Thick Volume

This is especially significant for persons who are shorter. You want to be able to sit up straight in your chair while being able to place both of your feet level on the ground. If it is not an option for you, try placing a yoga block or a heavy book under your feet instead.

Garments that are easy on the body

In an ideal situation, you should aim to dress in comfortable attire that does not limit your range of motion. Please take off your shoes. It is up to you whether you practice with socks or without shoes on your feet.

How to Get Started with Chair Yoga Here Are the Steps to Take

Take Note of Your Position

To get started, sit in your chair in a straight and upright position without slouching or sagging. In yoga, posture is very essential, not because it affects one's beauty, but rather because slouching impairs deep breathing and may cause the spine to become compressed. Adjust your seating position so that your shoulders are in line with the top of your pelvis. Put your chin in a position where it is parallel to the floor. You should turn your head such that the top of it points toward the ceiling.

Pay Attention to How You Are Breathing
The majority of us breathe quickly without even being conscious of the fact that we are doing so. The best approach to breathe for your health is to take as few breaths as possible every minute, but to do it in a leisurely and deep manner, making use of as much of your lungs as you can.

Our lungs have a surface area that is comparable to that of a tennis court, yet we tend to think of them as being much smaller than they really are. Take a long, slow breath in through your nose, and then let it out through your mouth. Then, continue to take deep breaths in until you feel the expansion of your diaphragm.

Continue to deepen the breath until you can feel your collar bones lifting as you reach the peak of the inhalation. The next step is to let go of the breath as gradually as possible, focusing on releasing air from the uppermost part of the lungs to the lowermost part.

Make it a goal to provide the same amount of time to both the inhale and the exhalation if at all feasible. As soon as you notice that the pattern of your breath has begun to calm down, you are ready to start stretching. As you carry out these exercises, don't forget to keep your breathing under control.

Relaxing Chair Yoga Sequence: Seated Twist
Raise the balls of your feet while keeping your toes planted on the ground (or on your block or book, whichever you want).

Draw your thighs in toward one another. As you take a deep breath in, visualize your spine becoming longer as your lungs fill up with air. Exhale, and as you are doing so, gently move your torso to the right. While you are doing this, move your legs so that they are pointing to the left. While holding this twisted posture, take three to six slow, deep breaths and work on spreading your upper and lower bodies apart as much as you can. After then, bring yourself back to the middle by drawing a deep breath in. On the other side, perform this sitting twist in the opposite direction.

As you continue to do this stretch, you will notice that the tension and stiffness in your back begin to ease. It is recommended that you do it twice, first in one direction and then the other.

Chair yoga stretches for your legs to relax.
You should wrap the strap around your right foot and hold it there (or belt, or leash). While doing so, bring your right knee into proper alignment and extend your right leg forward. Raise your toes off the floor while keeping the heel of your right foot in contact with the ground. Put the bottom of your foot up against the strap, and use your arms to give the strap a little tug while doing so. It ought to feel like there's a stretch going on in the rear of your right leg.

If you want to take this stretch to the next level, exhale and bend your chest over your leg while maintaining your buttocks firmly planted on the chair seat. This will take you farther into the stretch. You should maintain your left leg bent and your left foot planted firmly on the ground as you extend your right leg. Take a deep breath in, and then gently stand back up. Turning around will help you stretch out your left leg.

Chair Yoga Shoulder Stretch for Those Who Prefer a Slower Pace
Put your right hand on the leash (or strap, or belt), and hold it there. To begin, bring your right arm up and out to the side. Bend your right elbow while you are placing your right hand behind your head or neck. In an ideal situation, the strap should now be dangling behind your back in a relaxed manner.

Bring your left elbow behind you and a little bit apart from the rest of your body.

Extend your left hand toward your lower back after you have reached the point where you can grasp the lower end of the strap with your left hand. It is important that you keep your head and body in a neutral position as you do this stretch.

While you are stretching, take three to six deep breaths in as you inhale. Imagine that you are giving a massage to the muscles in your body that are resisting this stretch by using your breathing as the instrument. Check to see if you can get your hands onto the strap closer together over time without causing your head or spine to circle. After you have finished relaxing into the stretch, bring both hands back to your lap while exhaling. After that, do the same thing on the other side.

You should feel free to repeat each stretch many times. Alternately, if you are at work, you should do each stretch once to avoid your muscles from becoming stiff and tight as a result of spending an excessive amount of time sitting motionless. After you have finished stretching in this way, be sure to return to your seat and remain motionless for a while.

Shut your eyes. Take notice of the different and more relaxed sensation that your muscles are experiencing. Note the shift in perspective that comes about in your outlook on life as well. As your internal equilibrium is readjusted, you should start to feel a greater sense of calm and stability inside yourself.

There Is No Such Thing as the "Right" or "Wrong" Kind of Yoga to Practice at Your Age

Many individuals avoid yoga because they feel they are "too old" to start practicing it at their current age. They observe from the sidelines, feeling tired and tense as they see a young woman in her 20s contorting herself into a pretzel. The complete antithesis of this is chair yoga. A lot of people believe that chair yoga is intended for those who have trouble moving about, so they dismiss the idea that it may benefit them. Both of these presumptions are incorrect. Yoga, which dates back thousands of years, is known to have several positive effects on both one's physical and mental health. It is a common misconception, despite the fact that yoga is becoming more popular, that certain styles of yoga are only suitable for people of certain age ranges. In point of fact, there is no such thing as the "wrong" or "right" way to practice yoga for a certain age group.

Yoga is a versatile and adaptable practice that may be adapted to your own requirements and capabilities, regardless of your age. It doesn't matter how old you are, how much yoga experience you have, or how your body feels now; there is a yoga practice that will be useful to you. There are an infinite number of possible combinations, ranging from gentle and restorative styles of yoga such as Hatha and Yin Yoga to more strenuous and physically demanding styles such as Ashtanga and Vinyasa.

It is essential to understand that age is nothing more than a number, and that there are no age limits to practice yoga. Taking into consideration your specific goals, physical capabilities, and any current medical issues is the single most important step in determining which style of yoga is going to be the most beneficial to you. If you are still recovering from an injury, for example, you may find that a less strenuous practice is more appropriate. If you want to improve both your strength and your flexibility, you could find that using a method that is more dynamic is more effective.

The key to identifying the kind of yoga that is most beneficial for you is to have an open mind and to experiment with a variety of yoga practices until you locate the one that suits your unique needs and preferences best. Because it is a practice that is maintained throughout one's life, yoga enables practitioners of any age to realize their full potential. Therefore, make the most of the many benefits that yoga has to offer while appreciating the challenge that it presents.

Conclusion

Seniors can benefit greatly from chair yoga, a moderate and convenient type of exercise. Without placing too much strain on their bodies, this style of yoga is intended to help seniors enhance their physical and emotional well-being. Seniors who practice chair yoga can increase their strength, flexibility, and balance as well as lower their stress levels. Chair yoga is an excellent alternative for seniors who may have limited mobility or who want a softer type of exercise because of its versatility. So chair yoga is a wonderful way to be active, healthy, and happy as you age, regardless of how long you've been a practitioner of yoga.

As a low-impact activity, chair yoga is perfect for seniors who might suffer from joint discomfort or other physical restrictions. Seniors can safely practice yoga while sitting on a chair since it offers stability and support, allowing them to do so without fear of falling or getting hurt. Additionally, the activity gives seniors a chance to interact with others, which can enhance their overall wellbeing and mental health.

A fun and engaging method for seniors to stay active and keep their bodies moving is to incorporate chair yoga into their daily routine. Chair yoga is a fantastic way for seniors to stay active, healthy, and engaged as they age because of its wide range of physical and mental benefits. Therefore, chair yoga is a fantastic option for seniors of all abilities, whether they want to improve their balance, lower their stress levels, or simply stay active.